BLS

Basic Life Support

Provider Handbook

By Dr. Karl Disque

AF812142

Satori Continuum Publishing
1810 E Sahara Ave. Suite 1507
Las Vegas, NV 89104

Printed in the United States of America

Educational Service Disclaimer

This Provider Handbook is an educational service provided by Satori Continuum Publishing. Use of this service is governed by the terms and conditions provided below. Please read the statements below carefully before accessing or using the service. By accessing or using this service, you agree to be bound by all of the terms and conditions herein.

The material contained in this Provider Handbook does not contain standards that are intended to be applied rigidly and explicitly followed in all cases. A health care professional's judgment must remain central to the selection of diagnostic tests and therapy options of a specific patient's medical condition. Ultimately, all liability associated with the utilization of any of the information presented here rests solely and completely with the health care provider utilizing the service.

Version 2021.01

TABLE of CONTENTS

CHAPTER 1

GENERAL CONCEPTS OF BASIC LIFE SUPPORT

According to the Centers for Disease Control (CDC), heart disease continues to be the leading cause of death in the United States and is responsible for over 600,000 deaths every year. Research continues to improve how we respond with life-saving techniques to emergencies. These techniques are based on the most current research and are organized into a systematic response called the Chain of Survival, which begins with Basic Life Support (BLS). The Chain of Survival provides the victim the best chance to receive the care needed and return to a healthy life.

The heart pumps blood through the lungs, where blood takes in oxygen and releases carbon dioxide. This blood then returns to the heart where it is pumped out to vital organs—the heart and brain—as well as the rest of the body. When the heart stops, blood flow stops, and the person quickly becomes unconscious. Without blood flow, the heart and the brain quickly become damaged due to lack of oxygen. The actions that make up BLS try to prevent or slow the damage until the cause of the problem can be corrected. BLS improves a person's chance of surviving until advanced care becomes available.

Taking the right action quickly and confidently can make the difference between life and death for a person dealing with cardiac arrest.

Keys for BLS:

- Quickly start the Chain of Survival.
- Deliver high-quality chest compressions to circulate oxygen to the brain and vital organs.
- Know when and how to use an Automated External Defibrillator (AED).
- Provide rescue breathing.
- Understand how to work with other rescuers as part of a team.
- Know how to treat choking.

INITIATING CHAIN OF SURVIVAL

Early initiation of BLS has been shown to increase the probability of survival for a person experiencing cardiac arrest. To increase the odds of surviving a cardiac event, the rescuer should follow the steps in the Adult Chain of Survival *(Figure 1)*.

Adult Chain of Survival

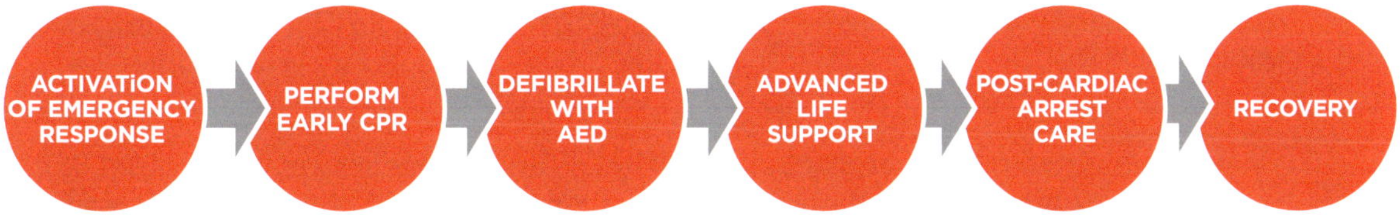

Figure 1

Emergencies in children and infants are not usually caused by the heart. Children and infants most often have breathing problems that trigger cardiac arrest. The first and most important step of the Pediatric Chain of Survival is prevention *(Figure 2)*.

Pediatric Chain of Survival

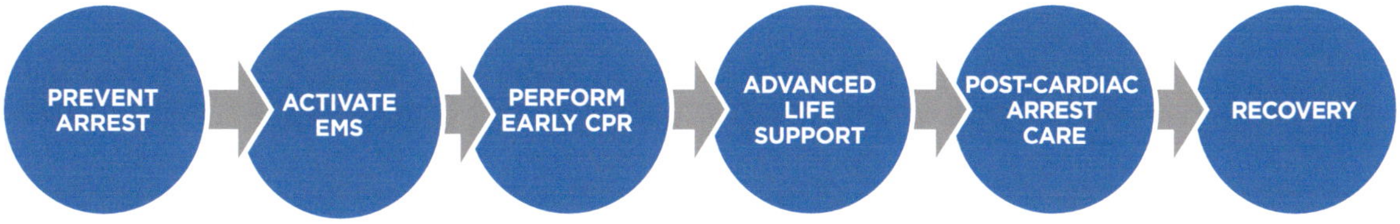

Figure 2

2020 BLS GUIDELINES CHANGES

Approximately every five years the International Liaison Committee on Resuscitation (ILCOR), updates the guidelines for CPR and ECC (Emergency Cardiac Care).

The content contained herein is based on the most recent ILCOR publications on BLS. Recommendations for adult basic life support (BLS) from the 2020 Guidelines for CPR and ECC include the following:

- The importance of early initiation of CPR by lay rescuers has been re-emphasized. The risk of harm to the patient is low if the patient is not in cardiac arrest. Bystanders should not be afraid to start CPR even if they are not sure whether the victim is breathing or in Cardiac Arrest.
- A sixth link, Recovery, was added to the Chains of Survival for both Pediatric and Adults.
- Care of the patient after return of spontaneous circulation (ROSC) requires close attention to oxygenation, blood pressure control, evaluation for percutaneous coronary intervention, targeted temperature management, and multimodal neuroprognostication.
- Because recovery from cardiac arrest continues long after the initial hospitalization, patients should have formal assessment and support for their physical, cognitive, and psychosocial needs.
- After a resuscitation, debriefing for lay rescuers, EMS providers, and hospital-based healthcare workers may be beneficial to support their mental health and well-being.
- Management of cardiac arrest in pregnancy focuses on maternal resuscitation, with preparation for early perimortem cesarean delivery if necessary to save the infant and improve the chances of successful resuscitation of the mother.

CHAPTER 2

BLS FOR ADULTS

BLS for adults focuses on doing several tasks simultaneously. In previous versions of BLS, the focus was primarily on one-rescuer CPR. In many situations, more than one person is available to do CPR. This simultaneous and choreographed method includes performing chest compressions, managing the airway, delivering rescue breaths, and using the AED, all as a team. By coordinating efforts, a team of rescuers can save valuable seconds when time lost equals damage to the heart and brain.

Simple Adult BLS Algorithm

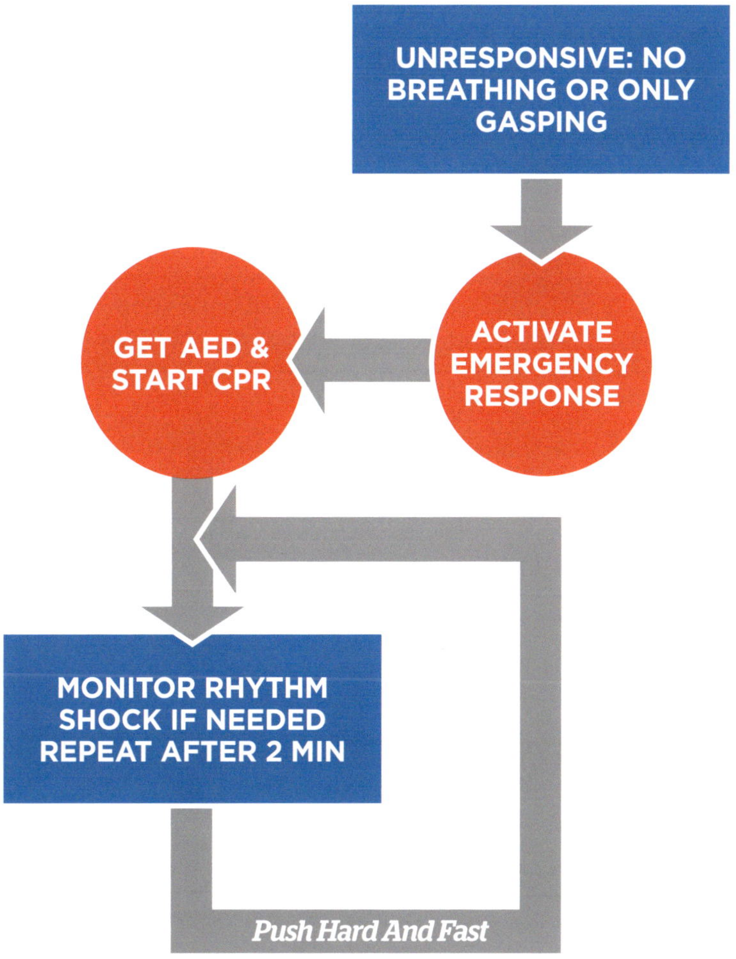

Figure 3

ONE-RESCUER BLS/CPR FOR ADULTS

Be Safe

- Make sure the scene is safe before proceeding.
- Move the person out of traffic.
- Move the person out of water and dry the person. (Drowning persons should be removed from the water and dried off; they should also be removed from standing water, such as puddles, pools, gutters, etc.)
- Be sure you do not become injured yourself.

Assess the Person

- Shake the person, tap their shoulder hard, and talk to them loudly.
- Check to see if the person is breathing. (Agonal breathing, which is occasional gasping and is ineffective, does not count as breathing.)

Call EMS

- Send someone for help or to call your emergency number and to get an AED.
- If alone, call for help while assessing for breathing and pulse. (The ILCOR emphasizes that cell phones are available everywhere now and most have a built-in speakerphone. Call for help without leaving the person.)

CPR

- Begin sets of compressions and rescue breaths.

Defibrillate

- Attach the AED pads when available.

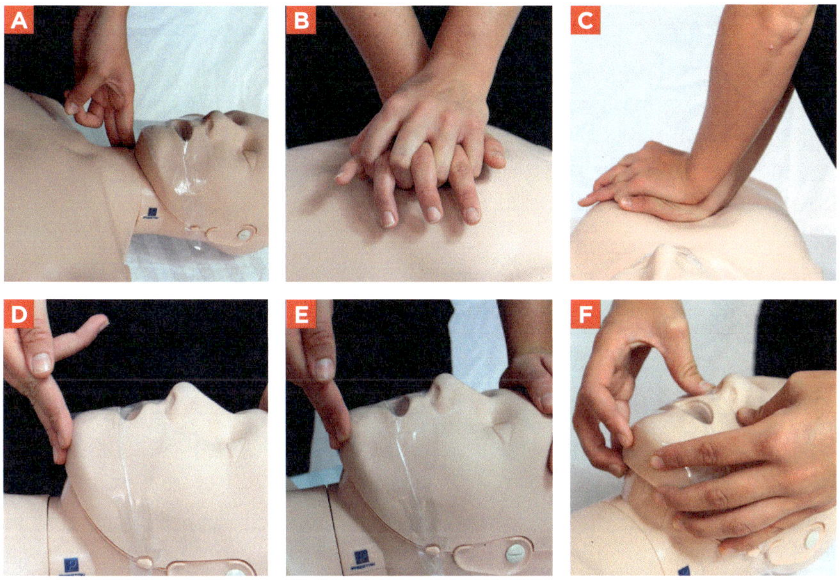

Figure 4

CPR STEPS

1. Check for the carotid pulse on the side of the neck *(Figure 4a)*. Keep in mind not to waste time trying to feel for a pulse; feel for no more than 10 seconds. If you are not sure you feel a pulse, begin CPR with a cycle of 30 chest compressions and two breaths.
2. Use the heel of one hand on the lower half of the sternum in the middle of the chest *(Figure 4b)*.
3. Put your other hand on top of the first hand *(Figure 4c)*.
4. Straighten your arms and press straight down *(Figure 4c)*. Compressions should be 2 to 2.4" (5 to 6 cm) into the person's chest and at a rate of 100 to 120 compressions per minute.
5. Be sure that between each compression you completely stop pressing on the chest and allow the chest wall to return to its natural position. Leaning or resting on the chest between compressions can keep the heart from refilling in between each compression and make CPR less effective.
6. After 30 compressions, stop compressions and open the airway by tilting the head and lifting the chin *(Figure 4d & 4e)*.
   a. Put your hand on the person's forehead and tilt the head back.
   b. Lift the person's jaw by placing your index and middle fingers on the lower jaw; lift up.
   c. Do not perform the head-tilt/chin-lift maneuver if you suspect the person may have a neck injury. In that case, the jaw-thrust is used.
   d. For the jaw-thrust maneuver, grasp the angles of the lower jaw and lift it with both hands, one on each side, moving the jaw forward. If their lips are closed, open the lower lip using your thumb *(Figure 4f)*.
7. Give a breath while watching the chest rise. Repeat while giving a second breath. Breaths should be delivered over one second.
8. Resume chest compressions. Switch quickly between compressions and rescue breaths to minimize interruptions in chest compressions.

TWO-RESCUER BLS/CPR FOR ADULTS

Many times there will be a second person available that can act as a rescuer. The ILCOR emphasizes that cell phones are available everywhere now and most have a built-in speakerphone. Direct the second rescuer to call 911 or Emergency Medical Services (EMS) without leaving the person while you begin CPR. This second rescuer can also find an AED while you stay with the person. When the second rescuer returns, the CPR tasks can be shared:

1. The second rescuer prepares the AED for use.
2. You begin chest compressions and count the compressions out loud.
3. The second rescuer applies the AED pads.
4. The second rescuer opens the person's airway and gives rescue breaths.
5. Switch roles after every five cycles of compressions and breaths. One cycle consists of 30 compressions and two breaths.
6. Be sure that between each compression you completely stop pressing on the chest and allow the chest wall to return to its natural position. Leaning or resting on the chest between compressions can keep the heart from refilling in between each compression and make CPR less effective. Rescuers who become tired may tend to lean on the chest more during compressions; switching roles helps rescuers perform high-quality compressions.
7. Quickly switch between roles to minimize interruptions in delivering chest compressions.
8. When the AED is connected, minimize interruptions of CPR by switching rescuers while the AED analyzes the heart rhythm. If a shock is indicated, minimize interruptions in CPR. Resume CPR as soon as possible.

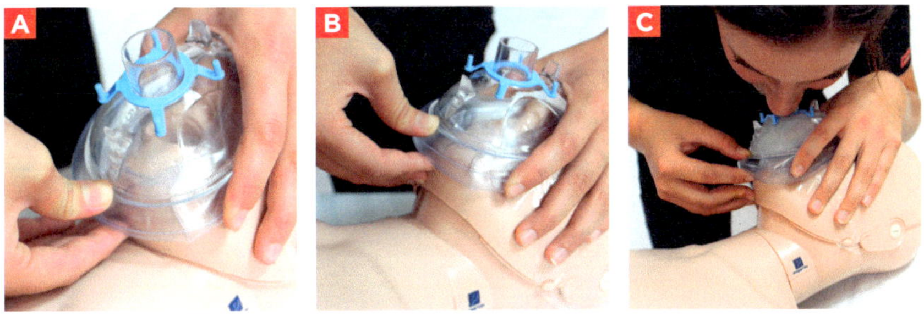

Figure 5

ADULT MOUTH-TO-MASK VENTILATION

In one-rescuer CPR, breaths should be supplied using a pocket mask, if available.

1. Give 30 high-quality chest compressions.
2. Seal the mask against the person's face by placing four fingers of one hand across the top of the mask and the thumb of the other hand along the bottom edge of the mask *(Figure 5a)*.
3. Using the fingers of your hand on the bottom of the mask, open the airway using the head-tilt/chin-lift maneuver. (Do not do this if you suspect the person may have a neck injury) *(Figure 5b)*.
4. Press firmly around the edges of the mask and ventilate by delivering a breath over one second as you watch the person's chest rise *(Figure 5c)*.

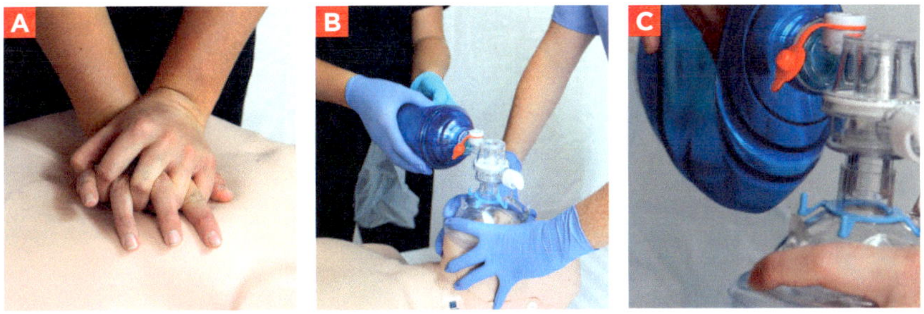

Figure 6

ADULT BAG-MASK VENTILATION IN TWO-RESCUER CPR

If two people are present and a bag-mask device is available, the second rescuer is positioned at the victim's head while the other rescuer performs high-quality chest compressions. Give 30 high-quality chest compressions.

1. Deliver 30 high-quality chest compressions while counting out loud *(Figure 6a)*.
2. The second rescuer holds the bag-mask with one hand using the thumb and index finger in the shape of a "C" on one side of the mask to form a seal between the mask and the face, while the other fingers open the airway by lifting the person's lower jaw *(Figure 6b)*.
3. The second rescuer gives two breaths over one second each as you watch the person's chest rise *(Figure 6c)*.
4. Practice using the bag-valve-mask; it is essential to forming a tight seal and delivering effective breaths.

Adult BLS Algorithm

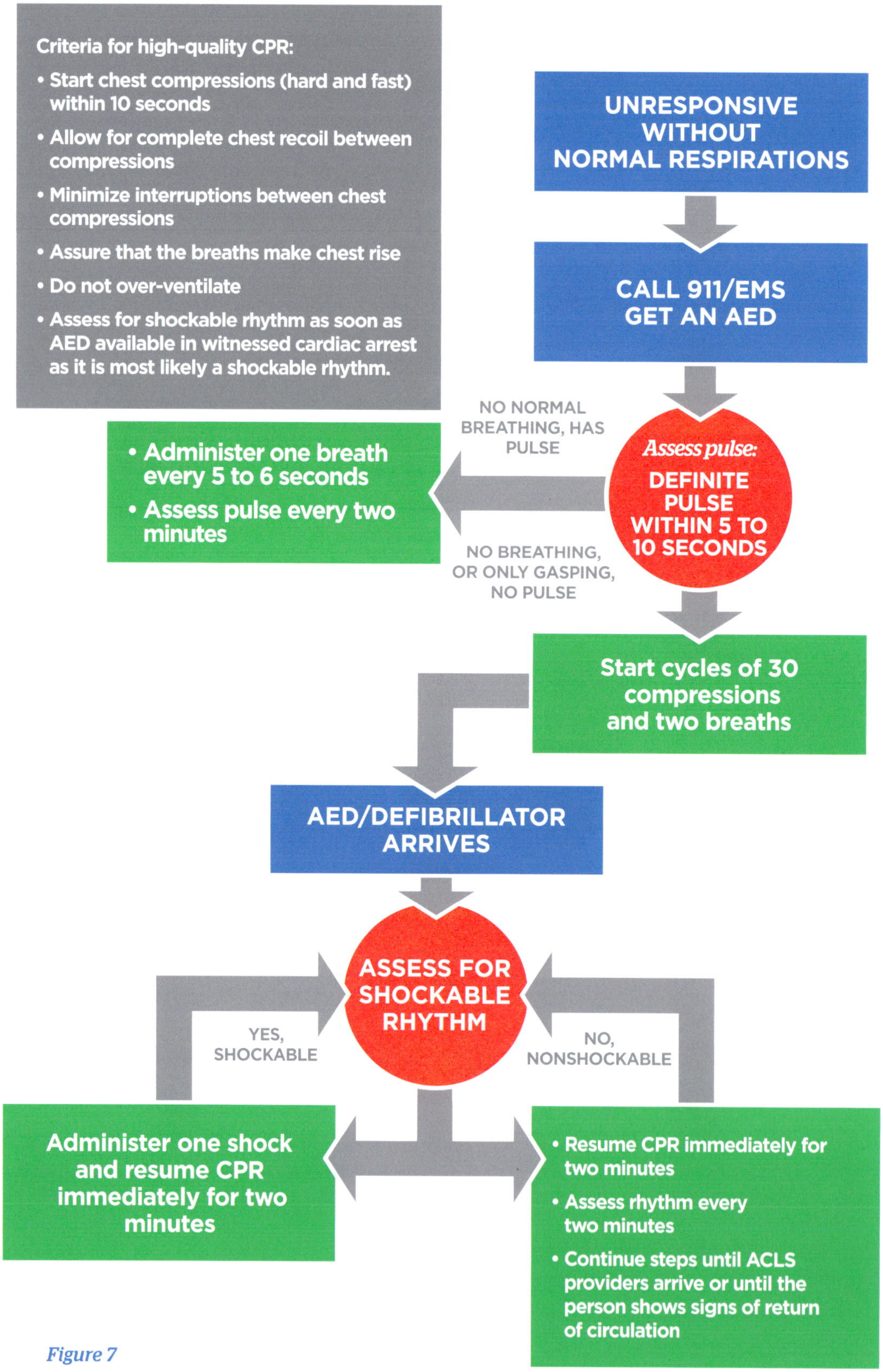

Figure 7

SELF-ASSESSMENT FOR ADULT BLS

1. A 65-year-old male is on a short ladder changing a light and suddenly collapses. He is unresponsive. What is the next step?
   a. Call 911/EMS.
   b. Begin CPR.
   c. Begin mouth-to-mouth ventilation.
   d. Check pulse.
2. What method should be used to open his airway in the case above?
   a. Chin-lift
   b. Jaw thrust
   c. Head-tilt/chin-lift
   d. Head-tilt
3. CPR is initiated and the person's pulse returns, but he is not breathing. What ventilation rate should be used for this person?
   a. 6-8 breaths per minute
   b. 10-12 breaths per minute
   c. 18-20 breaths per minute
   d. Depends on his color

ANSWERS

1. A
   Initiation of the Chain of Survival, which is to call 911/EMS, is the first step in the treatment of this person.
2. B
   The jaw thrust is the maneuver of choice to open this patient's airway given the concern of a fall and potential for traumatic injuries.
3. B
   Most experts recommend a ventilation rate of 10-12 breaths per minute for adults.

CHAPTER 3

USE OF AUTOMATED EXTERNAL DEFIBRILLATOR

Ventricular fibrillation, caused by disorganized electrical activity in the main pumping chambers of the heart, is a common cause of cardiac arrest. The treatment for ventricular fibrillation is defibrillation or the delivery of an electric shock to the heart through the person's chest wall. This shock attempts to stop the disorganized electrical activity and allow the heart's normal rhythm to resume.

The automated external defibrillator (AED) is a device that recognizes ventricular fibrillation and other dysrhythmias and delivers an electric shock at the right time. The AED has become a common sight in public buildings. The AED is nearly foolproof and will not allow you to make a mistake. It is safe for anyone to use. In a witnessed cardiac arrest, where the person is observed to suddenly collapse, the most common cause is likely to be ventricular fibrillation and a defibrillator should analyze the person's cardiac rhythm as soon as possible.

Using the team concept, one rescuer should coordinate all available rescuers so that one rescuer performs chest compressions while the second rescuer prepares the AED for use. Although there are many different brands of AEDs, all are utilized in a similar way. Be sure to move the person and yourself to a safe place before using the AED. Electricity and water can be lethal when combined. Ensure that the person is not wet (quickly wipe dry) or in close proximity to water before using the AED. It is safe to use an AED if the person is lying in snow. If the person has an implanted device, such as a pacemaker, you will see a bulge over their chest. Place the defibrillator pads as close to the correct position as possible without being directly over the device. For persons with medication patches, remove the patch, wipe the skin dry, and apply the AED pad.

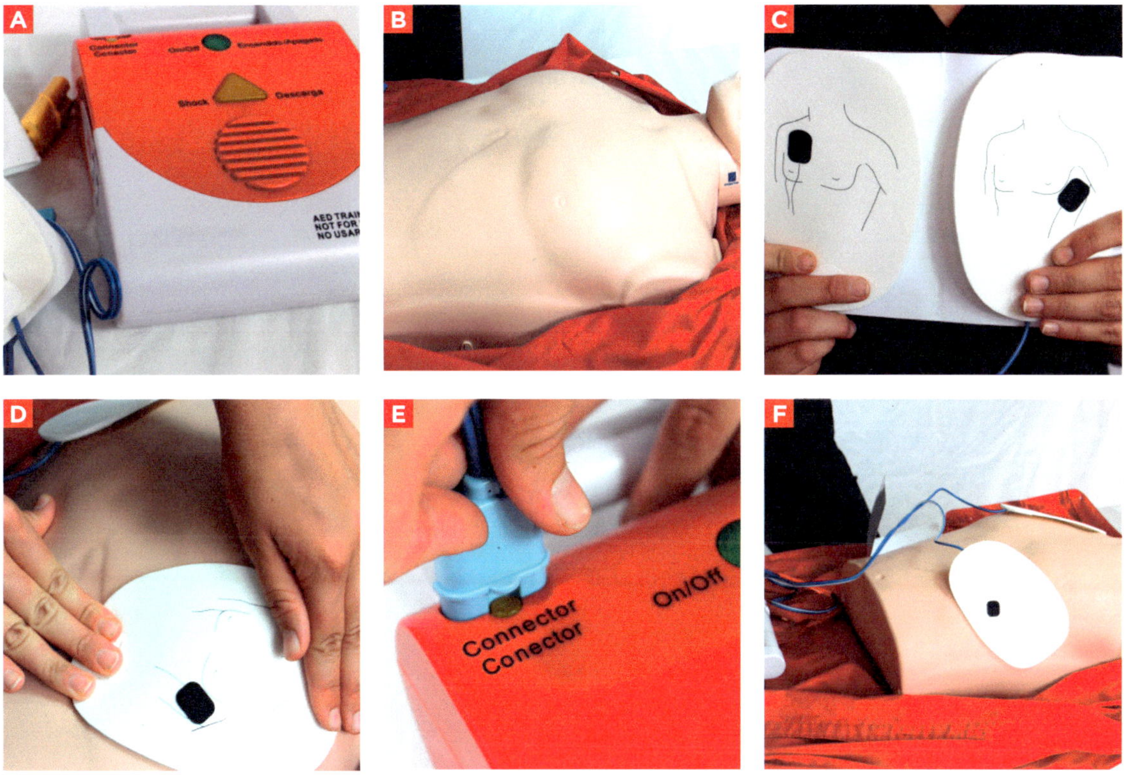

Figure 8

AED STEPS

1. Retrieve the AED *(Figure 8a)*.
   a. Open the case.
   b. Turn on the AED.
2. Expose the person's chest *(Figure 8b)*.
   a. If wet, dry chest.
   b. Remove medication patches.
3. Open the AED pads *(Figure 8c)*.
   a. Peel off backing.
   b. Check for pacemaker or internal defibrillator.
4. Apply the pads *(Figure 8d)*.
   a. Apply one pad on upper right chest above the breast.
   b. Apply the second pad on lower left chest below the armpit.
5. Ensure the wires are attached to the AED box *(Figure 8e)*.
6. Move away from the person *(Figure 8f)*.
   a. Stop CPR.
   b. Clear the person to make sure no one is touching any part of the victim.

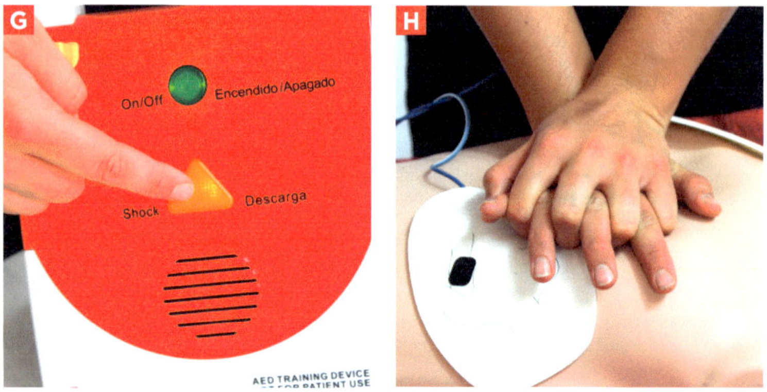

Figure 8

7. Let AED analyze the rhythm.
8. If AED message reads "Check Electrodes," then:
   a. Ensure electrodes make good contact.
   b. If chest is hairy, pull off pad and replace it.
9. If AED message reads "Shock,"
   a. Be sure the person is "clear" by making sure no one is touching them.
   b. Press and hold the "shock" button until the AED delivers the shock *(Figure 8g)*.
10. Resume CPR for two minutes starting with chest compressions *(Figure 8h)*.
11. Repeat steps 1 to 10.

SELF-ASSESSMENT FOR AED

1. What does AED stand for?
    a. Automatic Energy Delivery
    b. Automated External Device
    c. Automated External Defibrillator
    d. Autonomous Energy Defibrillator

A 49-year-old female suffers a witnessed cardiac arrest. She has a known cardiac history per her family.

2. You notice a bulge in the upper left chest under the skin. There is a healed incision overlying that bulge. Which is true of AED use?
    a. AED cannot be used in this person.
    b. You should put a magnet over the bulge before using the AED.
    c. You should place pads over the bulge.
    d. You should avoid placing pads over the bulge.
3. The AED indicates "Shock." What is the next step?
    a. Clear the person and deliver the shock.
    b. Deliver two additional minutes of CPR before delivering the shock.
    c. Ventilate while shock is delivered.
    d. Assume error and do not deliver shock.
4. After delivering a shock, what is the next step in caring for this person?
    a. Reassess for a pulse.
    b. Do chest compressions only.
    c. Resume CPR starting with chest compressions.
    d. Do ventilation only.

ANSWERS

1. C

AED stands for Automated External Defibrillator.

2. D

This person has either a pacemaker or an automated implantable cardioverter-defibrillator (AICD). Avoid placing AED pads directly over these devices.

3. A

Clear the person and deliver the shock. Do not delay delivery of a shock to perform additional CPR. All responders should be clear of the person when a shock is delivered. Do not assume error or delay administration of a shock.

4. C

After delivery of a shock, two minutes of high-quality CPR is performed. Do not perform a rhythm or pulse check at this point.

CHAPTER 4

BLS FOR CHILDREN (1 TO PUBERTY)

Many similarities exist between the BLS guidelines for adults and children. Following are the main differences between the two:

- For children of all age groups, the compression to breaths ratio is 30:2 for one rescuer and 15:2 for two rescuers.
- The depth of compression may be different. For children, compress the chest at least one-third the depth of the chest. This may be less than two inches for small children (4 -5 cm) but will be approximately two inches for larger children (5 cm).
- If you are the only rescuer at the scene and find an unresponsive child, perform CPR for two minutes before you call EMS or before you go look for an AED. The ILCOR emphasizes that cell phones are available everywhere now, and most have a built-in speakerphone, so you can call EMS while being with the child.
- In children, primary cardiac events are not common. Cardiac arrest is most commonly preceded by respiratory problems. Survival rates improve with early intervention for respiratory problems. Remember that prevention is the first link in the Pediatric Chain of Survival.
- If you witness a cardiac arrest in a child, call EMS and get an AED as you would in the Adult BLS sequence.

ONE-RESCUER BLS FOR CHILDREN

If you are alone with a child at the scene, do the following:

1. Tap and talk loudly to the child to determine if they are responsive.
2. If the child does not respond and is not breathing (or only gasping), yell for help. If someone answers, send them to call 911/EMS and to get an AED.
3. Assess for breathing while simultaneously checking for the child's carotid pulse (on the side of the neck) or femoral pulse (on the inner thigh in the crease between their leg and groin) for 5 but no more than 10 seconds.
4. If you cannot feel a pulse (or if you are unsure), begin CPR by doing 30 compressions followed by two breaths. If you can feel a pulse but the pulse rate is less than 60 beats per minute, you should begin CPR. This rate is too slow for a child.
5. After doing CPR for about two minutes (usually about five cycles of 30 compressions and two breaths), and if other help has not arrived, call EMS while staying with the child. The ILCOR emphasizes that cell phones are available everywhere now and most have a built-in speakerphone. Get an AED if you know where one is.
6. Use and follow AED prompts when available while continuing CPR until EMS arrives or until the child's condition normalizes.

TWO-RESCUER BLS FOR CHILDREN

If you are not alone with a child at the scene, do the following:

1. Tap and talk loudly at the child to determine if they are responsive.
2. If the child does not respond and is not breathing (or if only gasping), have the second rescuer call 911/EMS and get an AED. (The ILCOR emphasizes that cell phones are available everywhere now and most have a built-in speakerphone, so you or the second rescuer can call 911/EMS without leaving the scene).
3. Assess for breathing while simultaneously checking for the child's carotid pulse (on the side of the neck) or femoral pulse (on the inner thigh in the crease between their leg and groin) for 5 but no more than 10 seconds.
4. If you cannot feel a pulse (or if you are unsure), begin CPR by doing 15 compressions followed by two breaths. If you can feel a pulse but the pulse rate is less than 60 beats per minute, you should begin CPR. This rate is too slow for a child
5. When the second rescuer returns, begin doing CPR by performing 15 compressions by one rescuer and two breaths by the second rescuer.
6. Use and follow AED prompts when available while continuing CPR until EMS arrives or until the child's condition normalizes.

Pediatric BLS Algorithm

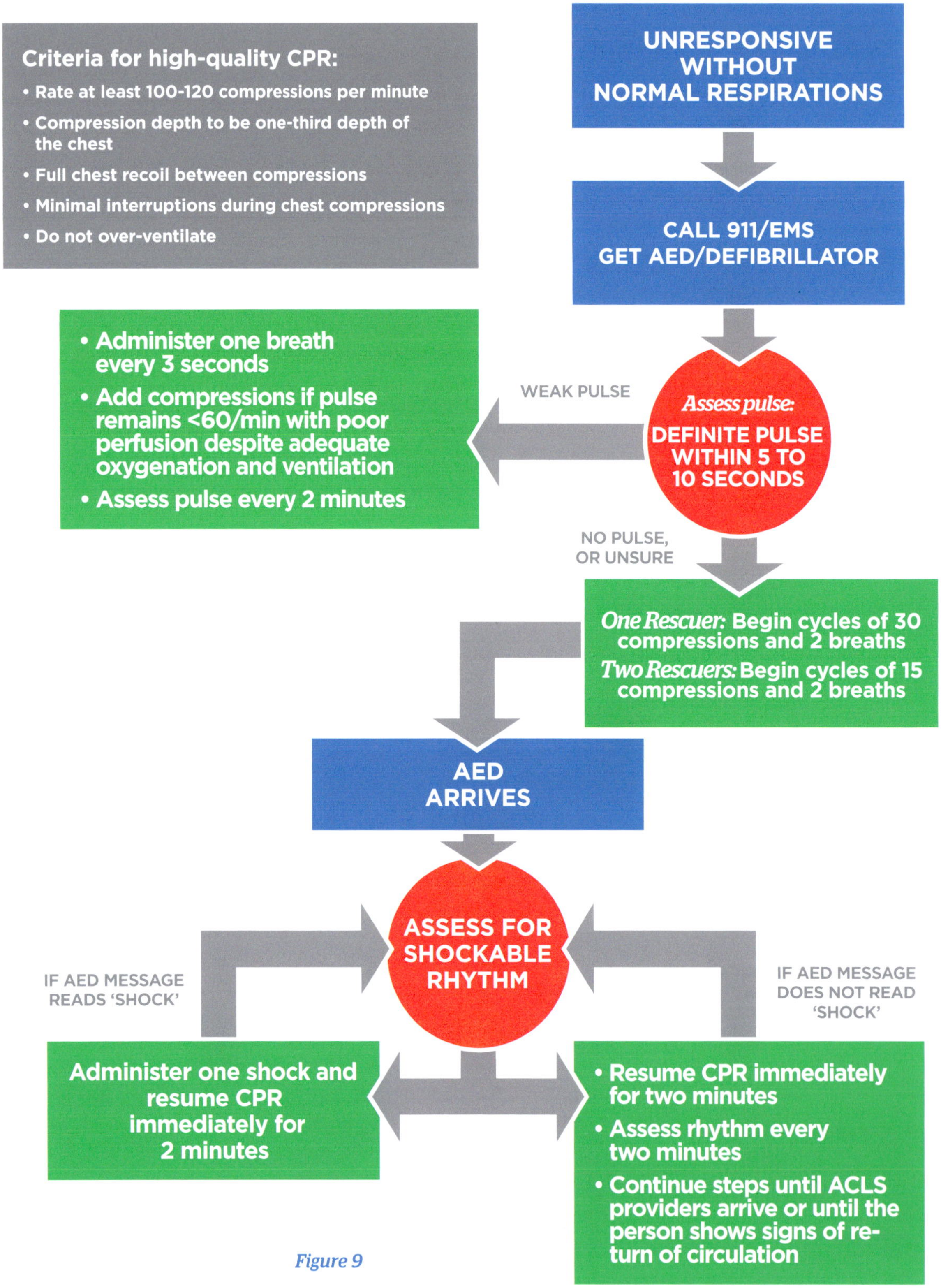

Figure 9

CHILD VENTILATION

If masks are available, they should be used in children as in adults; however, you must ensure the mask is the correct size for the child. The mask should cover the child's mouth and nose without covering the eyes or chin. You will not be able to get a good seal with a mask that is too big. As with an adult, use the head-tilt/chin-lift maneuver to open the child's airway. Each breath should last one second and should cause the child's chest to rise. As with an adult, avoid giving breaths too quickly, as this may result in distention of the stomach, vomiting, and possible aspiration of stomach contents.

Child Ventilation Algorithm

Figure 10

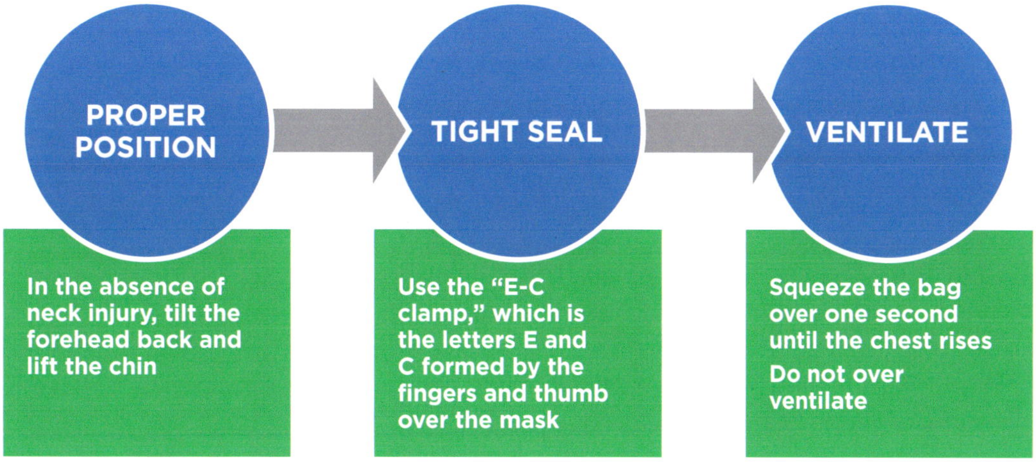

CHAPTER 5

BLS FOR INFANTS (0 TO 12 MONTHS)

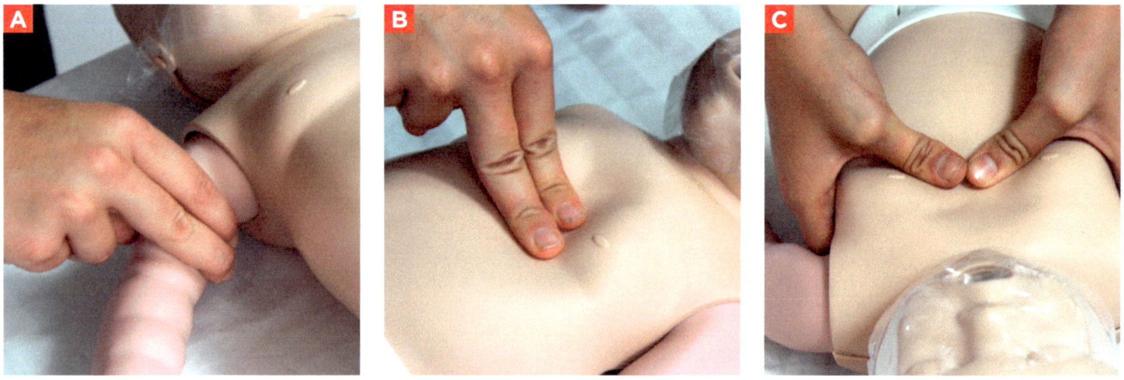

Figure 11

BLS for both children and infants is almost identical. Following are the main differences between BLS for children and BLS for infants:

- Check the pulse in the infant using the brachial artery on the inside of the upper arm between the infant's elbow and shoulder *(Figure 11a)*.
- During CPR, compressions can be performed on an infant using two fingers *(Figure 11b)*, if only one rescuer; or with two thumb-encircling hands *(Figure 11c)*, if there are two rescuers and rescuer's hands are big enough to go around the infant's chest.
- Compression depth should be one-third of the chest depth; for most infants, this is about 1.5 inches (4 cm).
- If you are the only rescuer at the scene and find an unresponsive infant, perform CPR for two minutes before calling 911/EMS or using an AED.
- In infants, primary cardiac events are not common. Usually, cardiac arrest will be preceded by respiratory problems. Survival rates improve when you intervene with respiratory problems as early as possible. Remember that prevention is the first step in the Pediatric Chain of Survival.
- If you witness a cardiac arrest in an infant, call 911/EMS and get an AED as you would in the BLS sequence for adults or children.

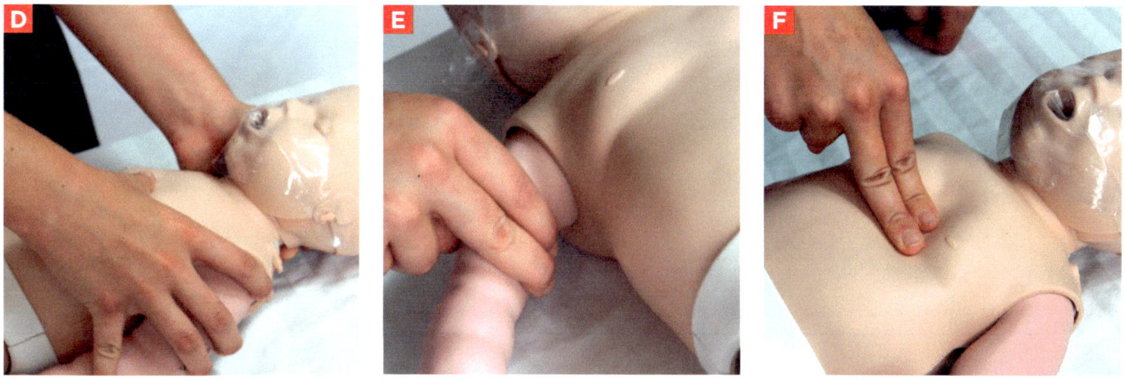

Figure 11

ONE-RESCUER BLS FOR INFANTS

If you are alone with the infant at the scene, do the following:

1. Tap the heel of their foot and talk loudly at the infant to determine if they are responsive.
2. Assess if they are breathing *(Figure 11d)* while simultaneously checking for the infant's brachial pulse for 5 but no more than 10 seconds *(Figure 11e)*. If the infant does not respond and is not breathing (only gasping), yell for help.
3. If someone responds, send the second rescuer to call 911/EMS and get an AED. (The ILCOR emphasizes that cell phones are available everywhere now and most have a built-in speakerphone, so rescuers do not have to leave the scene.)
4. If you cannot feel a pulse (or if you are unsure), begin CPR by doing 30 compressions followed by two breaths. If you can feel a pulse but the rate is less than 60 beats per minute, begin CPR. This rate is too slow for an infant. To perform CPR on an infant, do the following:
    a. Be sure the infant is face-up on a hard surface.
    b. Using two fingers, perform compressions in the center of the infant's chest *(Figure 11f)*; do not press on the end of the sternum as this can cause injury to the infant.
    c. Compression depth should be about 1.5 inches (4 cm) and 100-120 compressions per minute.
5. Perform CPR for about two minutes (using cycles of 30 compressions and two breaths). If help has not arrived, call 911/EMS and get an AED.
6. Use and follow AED prompts when available while continuing CPR until EMS arrives or until the infant's condition normalizes.

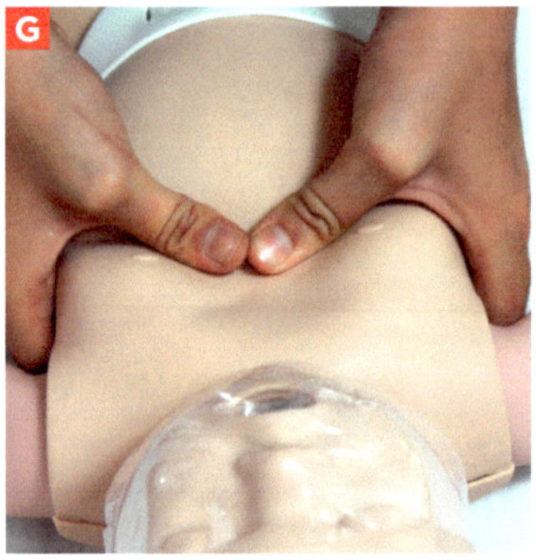

Figure 11

TWO-RESCUER BLS FOR INFANTS

If you are not alone with the infant at the scene, do the following:

1. Tap the bottom of their foot and talk loudly at the infant to determine if they are responsive.
2. If the infant does not respond, have the second rescuer call 911/EMS and get an AED. (The ILCOR emphasizes that cell phones are available everywhere now and most have a built-in speakerphone, so you can call while at the scene.)
3. Assess if they are breathing while simultaneously feeling for the infant's brachial pulse for 5 but no more than 10 seconds.
4. If you cannot feel a pulse (or if you are unsure), begin CPR by doing 15 compressions followed by two breaths. If you can feel a pulse but the rate is less than 60 beats per minute, begin CPR. This rate is too slow for an infant.
5. When the second rescuer returns, begin CPR by performing 15 compressions by one rescuer and two breaths by the second rescuer. If the second rescuer can fit their hands around the infant's chest, perform CPR using the two thumb-encircling hands method *(Figure 11g)*. Do not press on the bottom end of the sternum as this can cause injury to the infant.
6. Compressions should be approximately 1.5 inches (4 cm) deep and at a rate of at least 100-120 per minute.
7. Use and follow AED prompts when available while continuing CPR until EMS arrives or until the infant's condition normalizes.

CHAPTER 6

AED FOR CHILDREN AND INFANTS

An AED can be used on children and infants and should be used as early as possible for the best chance of improving the chance of survival. Check the AED when it arrives at the scene. Pediatric pads should be used if the person is less than eight years old or less than 55 pounds (25 kg). Standard (adult) pads may be used if pediatric pads are not available. If using standard (adult) pads, do not let the pads touch. For infants less than a year old, a manual defibrillator should be used if available. If a manual defibrillator is not available, an AED may be used. Some AEDs have a switch that can be set to deliver a pediatric shock. If available, turn the switch on when using on children younger than eight years old. If the AED cannot deliver a pediatric shock, an adult shock should be given. It is important to remember an electric shock may be the treatment for a fatal heart rhythm.

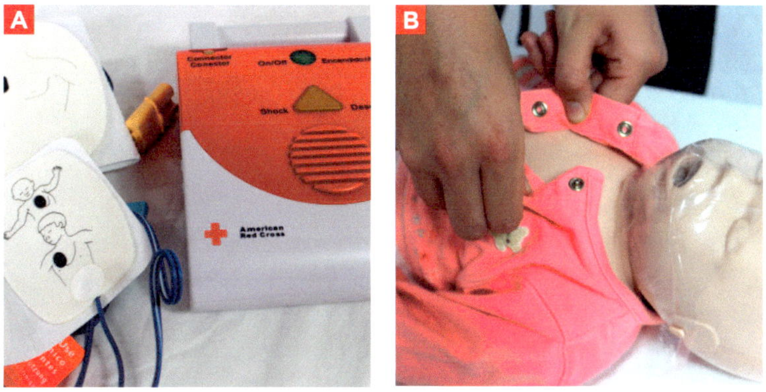

Figure 12

AED STEPS FOR CHILDREN AND INFANTS

1. Retrieve the AED *(Figure 12a)*.
   a. Open the case.
   b. Turn on the AED.
2. Expose the person's chest *(Figure 12b)*.
   a. If wet, dry the chest.
   b. Remove any medication patches.

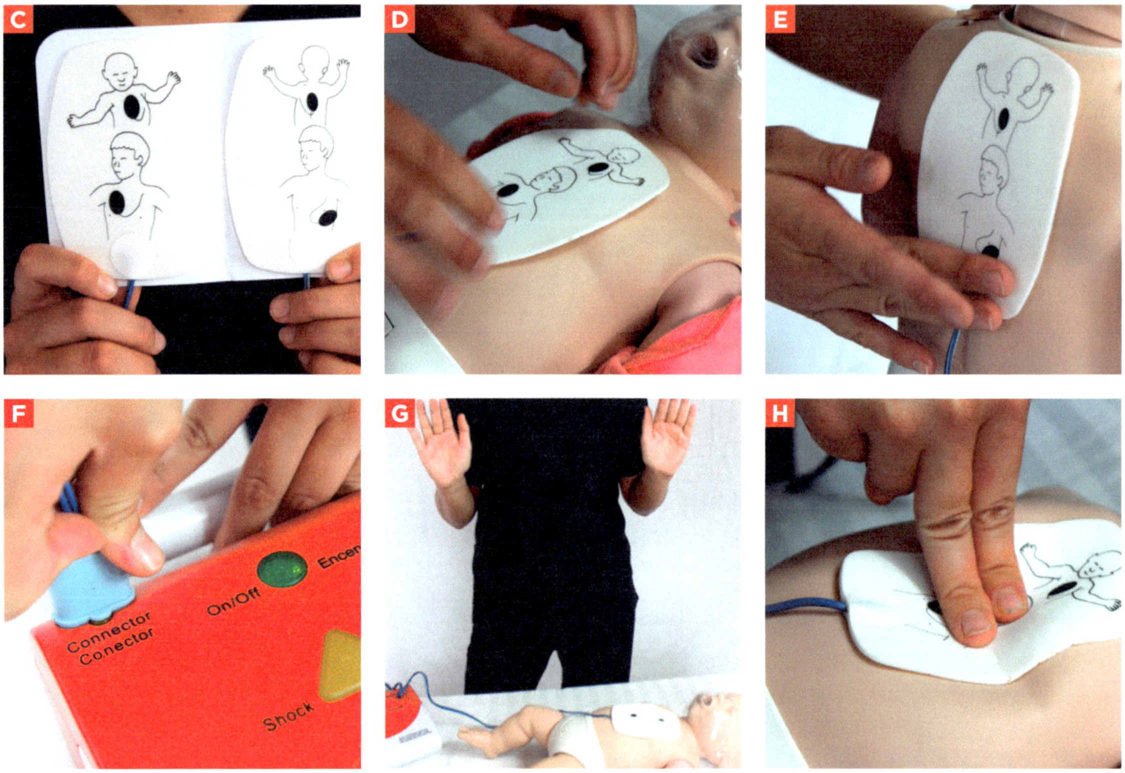

Figure 12

3. Open the Pediatric AED pads *(Figure 12c)*.
   a. Peel off backing.
   b. Check for pacemaker or implanted defibrillator.
4. Apply the pads *(Figure 12d)*.
   a. Apply one pad on the upper right chest above the breast. For infants, apply on front of chest
   b. Apply the second pad on lower left chest below the armpit. For infants, apply second pad to back *(Figure 12e)*.
5. Ensure wires are attached to the AED box *(Figure 12f)*.
6. Move away from the child *(Figure 12g)*.
   a. Stop CPR.
   b. Instruct others not to touch the person.
7. Let AED analyze the rhythm.
8. If AED message reads "Check Electrodes," then:
   a. Ensure electrodes make good contact *(Figure 12f)*.
9. If AED message reads "Shock," then:
   a. Press and hold flashing shock button until shock is delivered.
10. Resume CPR for two minutes starting with chest compressions *(Figure 12h)*.
11. Repeat steps 1-10.

SELF-ASSESSMENT FOR AED

1. What age is considered an infant for BLS purposes?
    a. Under one year
    b. Two years
    c. Three years
    d. Four years

2. Why are ventilations delivered to a pediatric arrest victim before seeking assistance in single-rescuer scenarios?
    a. 911/EMS response times are generally slow.
    b. The parents are often nearby.
    c. Most pediatric cardiac arrests are due to respiratory arrest.
    d. The use of an AED is contraindicated in pediatrics.

You are a daycare provider and find a 3-year-old child who is unresponsive. She had laid down for a nap because she was not feeling well. When you checked on her, she was not breathing and appeared blue. You are by yourself.

3. What is the first step in managing this case?
    a. Give back blows.
    b. Do a blind finger sweep.
    c. Call 911/EMS.
    d. Deliver two minutes of CPR.

4. The child begins to breathe spontaneously at a rate of 18. Her pulse is 50. What is the next step?
    a. Give faster rescue breaths.
    b. Do carotid massage.
    c. Begin CPR starting with chest compressions.
    d. Monitor breathing.

ANSWERS

1. A
   For BLS definitions, an infant is under one year of age. A child is 1 year of age to puberty. The BLS algorithms place children over the age of adolescence into the adult category.

2. C
   Respiratory arrest is the most common cause of cardiac arrest in children. Restoration of oxygen delivery can be life-saving and prevent a cardiac arrest.

3. D
   If you are alone, unwitnessed arrest in a child requires two minutes of CPR before calling 911/EMS. If assistance is available, send them to call 911/EMS while you begin CPR.

4. C
   CPR should be initiated for pediatrics with a heart rate (pulse) that is 60 or less.

CHAPTER 7

AIRWAY MANAGEMENT

Until an advanced airway is inserted, the rescue team should use mouth-to-mouth, mouth-to-mask, or bag-mask ventilation. An advanced airway (supraglottic airway, laryngeal mask airway, or endotracheal tube) provides a more stable way of providing breaths and should, therefore, be inserted as early as possible in a resuscitation effort. Once an advanced airway is in place, the compression to breath ratio should be adjusted as noted below *(Table 1)*.

The compression rate for all persons is always 100-120 per minute.

COMPRESSION TO BREATH RATIO	NO ADVANCED AIRWAY	ADVANCED AIRWAY
Adult	*30 compressions followed by two breaths*	*One breath every 6 seconds without pauses in compressions*
Child/Infant	*30 compressions followed by two breaths for one rescuer* *15 compressions followed by two breaths for two rescuers*	*One breath every 6 seconds without pauses in compressions* *One breath every 2-3 seconds (20-30 breaths per minute)*

Table 1

MOUTH-TO-MOUTH RESCUE BREATHING

When a pocket mask or bag-mask is not available, it may be necessary to give mouth-to-mouth breaths during CPR. Mouth-to-mouth breathing is very effective in delivering oxygen into the person's lungs without putting the rescuer at a high level of risk. The rescuer's exhaled air contains approximately 17% oxygen and 4% carbon dioxide. This is in contrast to the 100% oxygen available with ventilation with 100% high flow oxygen and the 21% oxygen that is available in room air that we breathe.

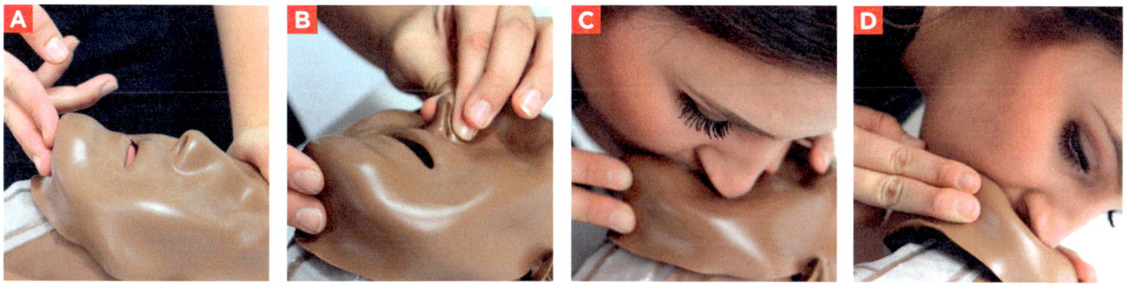

Figure 13

ADULTS AND OLDER CHILDREN MOUTH-TO-MOUTH

Do not give breaths too rapidly or too forcefully. Doing this may cause air to be forced into the stomach, resulting in distention and less room for lung expansion. It may also cause vomiting.

To deliver mouth-to-mouth breaths, do the following:

1. Open the airway using the head-tilt/chin-lift maneuver *(Figure 13a)*.
2. Pinch the person's nose closed with your hand on the person's head *(Figure 13b)*.
3. Create a seal when using your lips to surround the person's mouth *(Figure 13c)*.
4. Blow into the person's mouth for one full second and watch for chest to rise *(Figure 13d)*. Tilt the victim's head further back if the chest does not rise.
5. Give an additional breath for over one second.
6. If you cannot see the chest rise in two breaths, continue giving chest compressions.

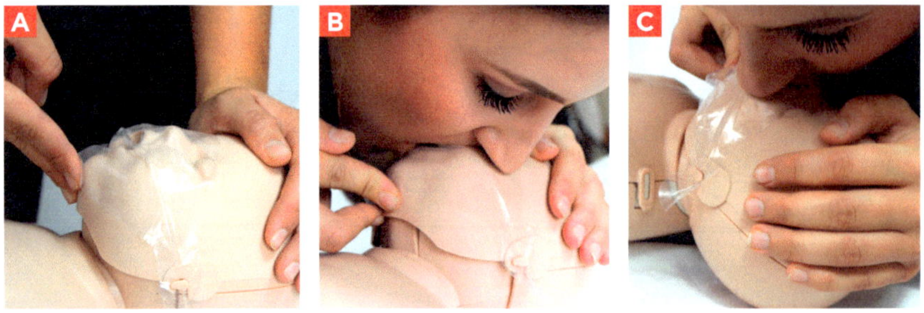

Figure 14

INFANTS MOUTH-TO-MOUTH/NOSE

When performing rescue breathing on an infant, the rescuer should cover the infant's mouth and nose when possible and do the following:

1. Open the airway using the head-tilt/chin-lift maneuver *(Figure 14a)*. Be sure not to hyper-extend the neck. Aim for a neutral position.
2. Create a seal using your lips to surround the infant's nose and mouth *(Figure 14b)*.
3. Gently blow into the infant's nose and mouth for one second *(Figure 14c)*. Keep in mind that an infant's lungs are smaller than an adult's and need a smaller volume of air. Watch for the infant's chest to rise. If you cannot see the chest rise, re-adjust the tilt of their head.
4. Give an additional breath and watch for the infant's chest to rise. If unable to cover both mouth and nose entirely with your mouth, use the following method for rescue breathing:
    a. Open the airway using the head-tilt/chin-lift maneuver.
    b. Pinch the infant's nose closed.
    c. Create a seal using your lips to surround the infant's mouth.
    d. Gently blow into the infant's mouth for one second.
    e. Give an additional breath and watch for the chest to rise.

RESCUE BREATHING

In many cases, cardiac arrest is preceded by respiratory arrest. Therefore, it is important to be able to recognize respiratory issues in order to take steps to prevent cardiac arrest.

When a person of any age has a pulse but is not breathing (or is not breathing well), immediately open the airway using the head-tilt/chin-lift maneuver and begin rescue breathing. See *Table 2* for details on rescue breathing.

Table 2

<table>
<tr><th>AGE GROUP</th><th>HOW OFTEN</th><th>BREATHS PER MINUTE</th><th>DURATION</th><th>EVALUATION</th></tr>
<tr><td>Adult</td><td>Every 6 seconds</td><td>10 to 12 breaths per minute</td><td rowspan="2">Each breath should last one second</td><td rowspan="2">Check for chest rise and breathing;
Check pulse and begin CPR if necessary</td></tr>
<tr><td>Child/Infant</td><td>One rescuer:
Every 6 seconds
Two rescuers:
Every 2 to 3 seconds</td><td>One rescuer:
10 to 12 breaths per minute
Two rescuers:
20 to 30 breaths per minute</td></tr>
</table>

CHAPTER 8

RELIEF OF CHOKING

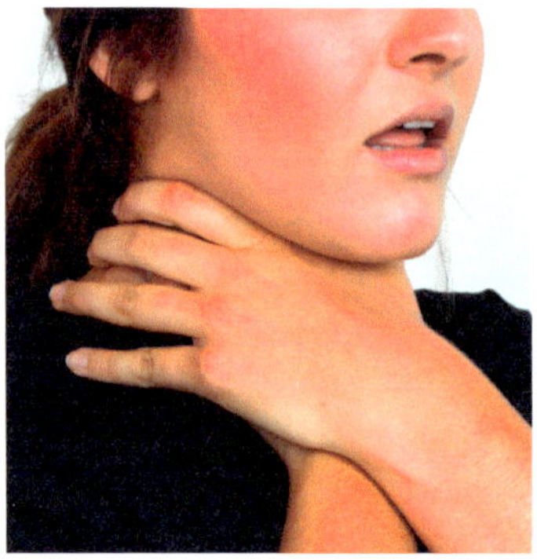

Figure 15

Choking is a common preventable cause of cardiac arrest. The correct response for a choking person depends on the degree of airway obstruction, whether the person is responsive or not, and the age of the person. See *Table 3* for rescue actions for choking in adult and children.

Choking In Adults And Children

DEGREE OF OBSTRUCTION	PERSON'S RESPONSE	RESCUER'S ACTION
Mild Obstruction	• *breathing but may also be wheezing* • *coughing and making noise*	• *stay with the person and try to keep them calm* • *encourage them to cough* • *call 911/EMS if the person seems to be getting worse*
Severe Obstruction	• *clutching the neck (universal sign of choking: figure 15)* • *weak or no cough* • *unable to make noise or talk; may make high-pitched noise* • *little or no breathing* • *may be cyanotic (blue around lips and fingertips)*	• *use abdominal thrusts to attempt to remove obstruction* • *call 911/EMS* • *begin BLS if the person becomes unresponsive*

Table 3

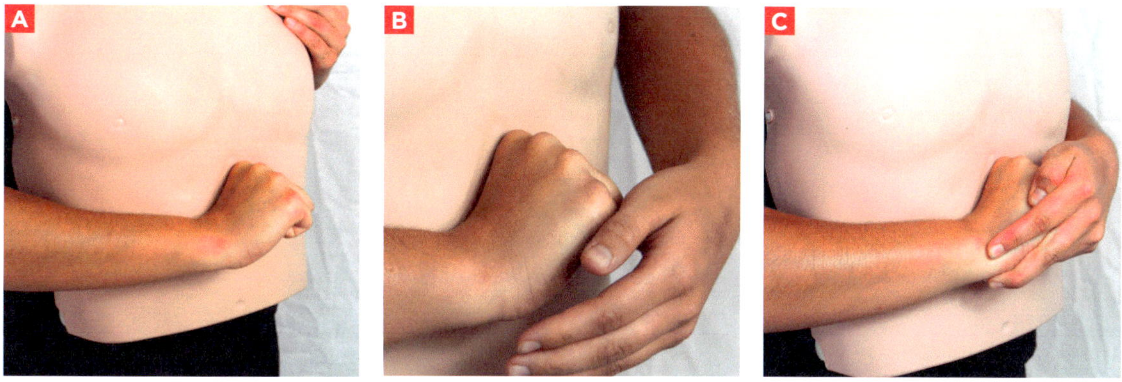

Figure 16: Abdominal Thrusts

If you can see a foreign object in the individual's mouth and can easily remove it, then do it. Watch and feel for breathing to begin. If the individual does not begin breathing, continue to provide CPR and rescue breaths until help arrives.

Abdominal Thrusts

These steps should only be used when a person is responsive and older than one year of age.

To properly perform abdominal thrusts, do the following:

1. Stand behind the responsive person. Wrap your arms around their waist under their ribcage.
2. Put the side of your fist above the person's navel in the middle of their belly. Do not press on the lower part of the sternum *(Figure 16a)*.
3. With your other hand, hold the first fist and press forcefully into the person's abdomen and up toward their chest *(Figure 16b and 16c)*.
4. Continue performing these thrusts until the obstruction is relieved or until the person becomes unresponsive.

Choking In Infants

DEGREE OF OBSTRUCTION	INFANT'S RESPONSE	RESCUER'S ACTION
Mild Obstruction	• *breathing but may also be wheezing* • *may be coughing and making noise*	• *stay with the infant and try to keep them calm* • *do not do a blind finger sweep* • *call 911/EMS if infant does not quickly clear the obstruction*
Severe Obstruction	• *weak or no cough* • *unable to make noise; may make high-pitched noise* • *little or no breathing* • *may be cyanotic (blue around lips and fingertips)*	• *use back blows/chest thrusts to attempt to remove obstruction* • *call 911/EMS* • *begin BLS if infant becomes unresponsive* • *assess if obstruction is visible; if so, remove it*

Table 4

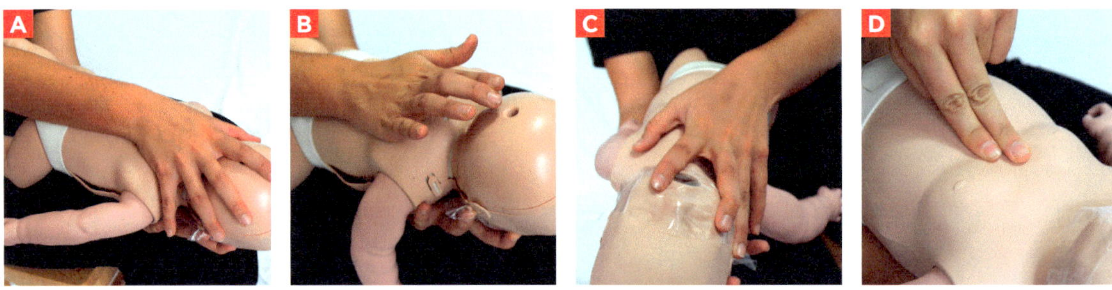

Figure 17

BACK BLOWS AND CHEST THRUSTS IN INFANTS

In a choking but responsive infant less than one-year-old, back blows and chest thrusts are used instead of abdominal thrusts. See *Table 4* for rescue actions for choking in infants. To provide back blows and chest thrusts, do the following:

1. Hold the infant in your lap.
2. Put the infant with their face down and their head lower than their chest; they should be resting on your forearm. Put your forearm on your thigh *(Figure 17a)*.
3. Support the infant's head and neck with your hand and be sure to avoid putting pressure on their throat.
4. Using the heel of your free hand, deliver five back blows between the infant's shoulder blades *(Figure 17b)*.
5. Using both hands and arms, turn the infant face up so they are now resting on your other arm; this arm should now be resting on your thigh *(Figure 17c)*.
6. Make sure the infant's head is lower than their chest.
7. Using the fingers of your free hand, provide up to five quick downward chest thrusts over the lower half of the breastbone *(Figure 17d)*. Perform one thrust every second.
8. If the obstruction is not relieved, turn the infant face down on your other forearm and repeat the process *(Figure 17b)*.
9. Continue doing these steps until the infant begins to breathe or becomes unresponsive.

SELF-ASSESSMENT FOR RELIEF OF CHOKING

A 21-year-old intoxicated college student turns blue and collapses while eating a hot dog at a bar.

1. What is most likely the cause?
    a. Cardiac arrest
    b. Alcohol poisoning
    c. Choking
    d. Drug ingestion
2. You assess that the student still has a pulse. What is the next step in managing this case?
    a. Begin CPR
    b. Open airway
    c. Apply AED
    d. Put in Recovery position
3. You are concerned that this student may have choked. What is the best method to clear an obstruction from the airway?
    a. Back blows
    b. Abdominal thrusts
    c. Start CPR
    d. Blind finger sweep

ANSWERS

1. C
   The color change suggests that he is choking. Patients who are intoxicated are at an increased risk of choking and aspirating food.
2. B
   After determining unresponsiveness and activating EMS, open his airway. The choking due to a hot dog being lodged in the airway must be dealt with first.
3. C
   If the choking person is unresponsive and already on the floor, begin CPR with chest compressions first.

CHAPTER 9

ADDITIONAL TOOLS

MEDICODE

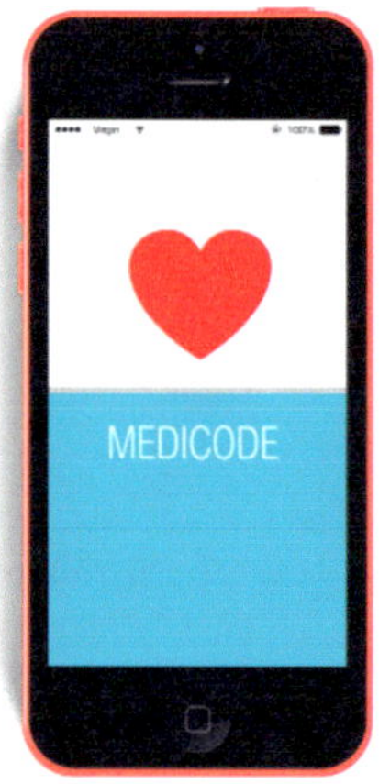

With MediCode, you no longer will have to carry a set of expandable cards with you at all times while at work. You will never have to waste valuable time in an emergency situation searching through multiple algorithms until you find the right one. All of the algorithms are now accessible from the palm of your hand, and you will be selecting your desired algorithm by memory in no time. Choose between multiple viewing options and easily share algorithms with co-workers and friends through email and social media.

To improve functionality and speed in obtaining your desired algorithm as quickly as possible in an emergency, they have been divided between BLS, ACLS, PALS, and CPR. All are accessible from the home screen.
The individual algorithms included in this app are:

- Basic Life Support (BLS)
- Advanced Cardiac Life Support (ACLS)
- Pediatric Advanced Life Support (PALS)
- Cardiopulmonary Resuscitation (CPR) AED, and First Aid

CERTALERT+

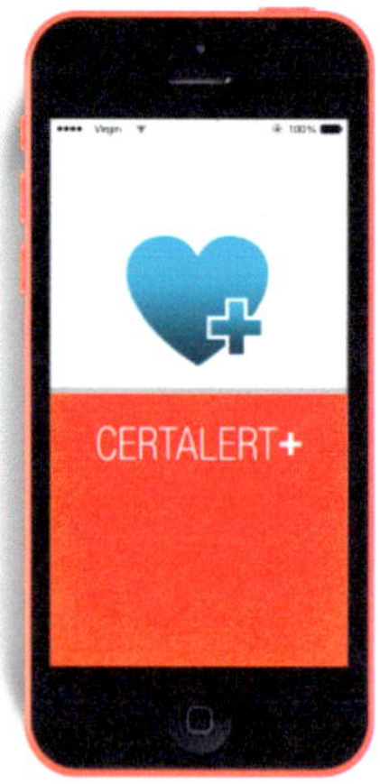

CertAlert+ is the perfect app to minimize a potential area of stress and distraction in your life. With CertAlert+, you will have all your licenses and certifications in one place anytime you need them. We will keep track and remind you when your expiration date approaches, and we will help you with your registration whenever possible.

With CertAlert+, you can:

- Compile all required licenses and certifications in one location.
- Take photos (front and back) of certification cards and licenses for simple reference.
- Record all expiration dates and store with ease.
- Choose when you want to be reminded of your approaching expiration dates.
- Send all license or certification information directly to your email after exporting from the app.
- Quick access to easily register for online certification and recertification courses.

CHAPTER 10

BLS REVIEW QUESTIONS

1. The 2020 ILCOR Guidelines for CPR changed the recommended compressions to ventilations ratio for Pediatrics to:
    a. 15:2 for all scenarios
    b. 30:2 for all scenarios
    c. 30:2 for 1 provider, then switch to 15:2 for 2 providers
    d. 15:2 for 1 provider, then switch to 30:2 for 2 providers
2. Critical characteristics of high-quality CPR include which of the following?
    a. Start chest compressions within 10 seconds of recognition of cardiac arrest
    b. Allow complete chest recoil after each compression
    c. Minimize interruptions of CPR
    d. All of the above
3. At what age is it preferable to use the pediatric AED pads?
    a. 8 years of age or older
    b. Less than 8 years of age
    c. 12 years of age or younger
    d. 18 years of age or younger
4. The compression to ventilation ratio for single rescuer giving CPR to an Adult is:
    a. 30:1
    b. 30:2
    c. 15:1
    d. 15:2
5. Where should you attempt to perform a pulse check in an adult?
    a. Brachial artery
    b. Carotid artery
    c. Popliteal artery
    d. Temporal artery
6. An AED can be used safely in all of the following situations except:
    a. Victim lying in the snow
    b. Victim with an implanted pacemaker
    c. Victim with a transdermal medication patch on
    d. Victim lying partially in water
7. The 6 steps in the Adult Chain of Survival include all of the following except:
    a. Early CPR
    b. Rapid defibrillation
    c. Use of cardiovascular medications
    d. Integrated post-cardiac arrest care

8. You are alone when you encounter a person in what appears to be cardiac or respiratory arrest. What are the first three steps you should take to stabilize the person? Check for danger, ___________, and send for help.

   a. Establish IV access
   b. Insert an advanced airway
   c. Check for response
   d. Start CPR

9. In both children and infants, two minutes of CPR should be given if:

   a. Witnessed cardiac arrest
   b. Unwitnessed collapse
   c. Witnessed choking incident
   d. Unresponsive victim with pulse and breathing

10. The proper steps for operating an AED are:

   a. Power on the AED, attach electrode pads, shock the person, and analyze the rhythm
   b. Power on the AED, attach electrode pads, analyze the rhythm, and shock the person
   c. Power on the AED, analyze the rhythm, attach electrode pads, and shock the person
   d. Power on the AED, shock the person, attach electrode pads, and analyze the rhythm

ANSWERS

1. C
   30:2 for 1 provider, then switch to 15:2 for 2 providers

2. D
   All of the above

3. B
   Less than 8 years of age, weighing 55 pounds (25 kg). Eight years old and older (to adult) use adult pads.

4. B
   30:2

5. B
   Carotid artery

6. D
   Victim lying partially in water

7. C
   Use of cardiovascular medications

8. C
   Check for response.

9. B.
   If you come across a child with unwitnessed collapse, perform 2 minutes of CPR if you are alone and can't call for help.

10. B
   Power on the AED, attach electrode pads, analyze the rhythm, and shock the person.

Who is the **Disque** Foundation?

The Disque Foundation was created for the sole purpose of empowering others to save lives! We do this by providing advanced healthcare education to underserved populations of the U.S. and the world through technology.

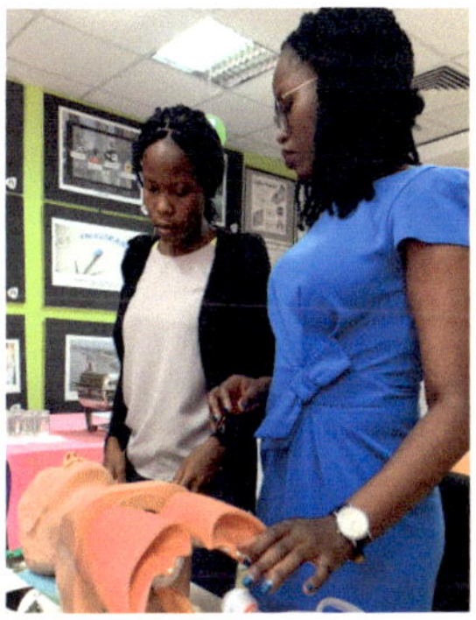
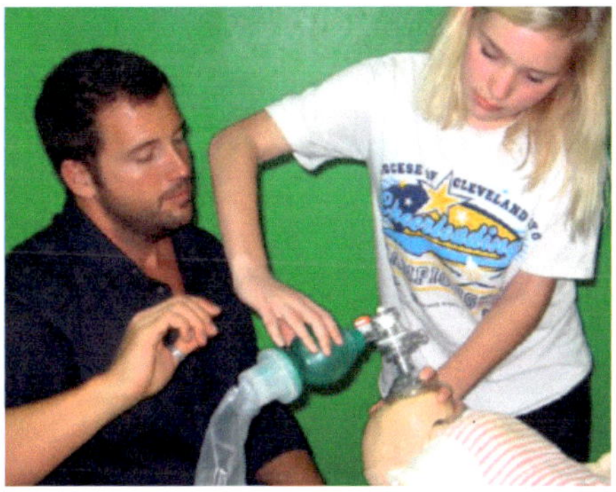
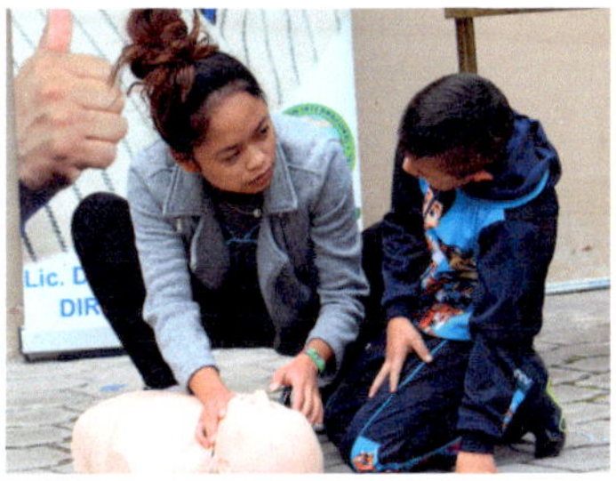
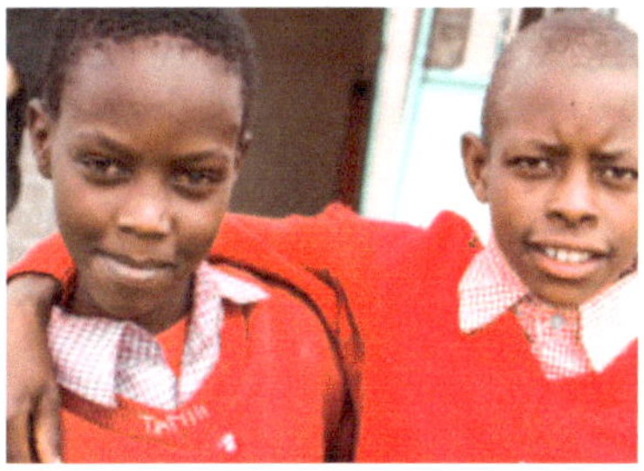

To fulfill this mission, we have created the Save a Life Initiative. We offer the world's first free life support training courses online through our partnership with SavealLife.com (Save a Life Certifications by NHCPS). Saving lives means giving others the chance to make a difference in the world. Our goal is to empower 10 million people with the ability to save a life by 2025.

How can I help?

Through the help of committed supporters like yourself, the Disque Foundation will have the ability to grow and expand our cause across the globe. Please help us by making a tax-deductible gift to the Disque Foundation. A donation of any size will help support our mission and your generous contribution will go directly to strengthening our efforts to empower others to save lives.

Donations can be made at **DisqueFoundation.org** or by mailing a check to:

Disque Foundation Donations Department
1609 W 100 S.
Brownstown, IN 47220
For more information, contact us at **info@disquefoundation.org**.

DISQUE™ FOUNDATION

Learn more at
DisqueFoundation.org

SaveaLife INITIATIVE™

The idea behind the Save a Life Initiative is simple – take the same advanced life-saving training we developed for health care providers, and give it to the underserved, at home and abroad. We work in conjunction with SaveaLife.com to fulfill its mission of advancing health care education to the underserved through advanced technology. When we put the knowledge, skills, and ability to perform CPR and other proven techniques in people's hands around the world, the power to save lives is possible.

Made in the USA
Monee, IL
05 November 2026

67988162R00024